HOLLY LARSEN

Live The Carnivore Diet Life

A beginner's guide to shed fat and end bloating, reduce aches and pains that limit your life, and gain the energy to get off the couch and move.

First edition

This book was professionally typeset on Reedsy.
Find out more at reedsy.com

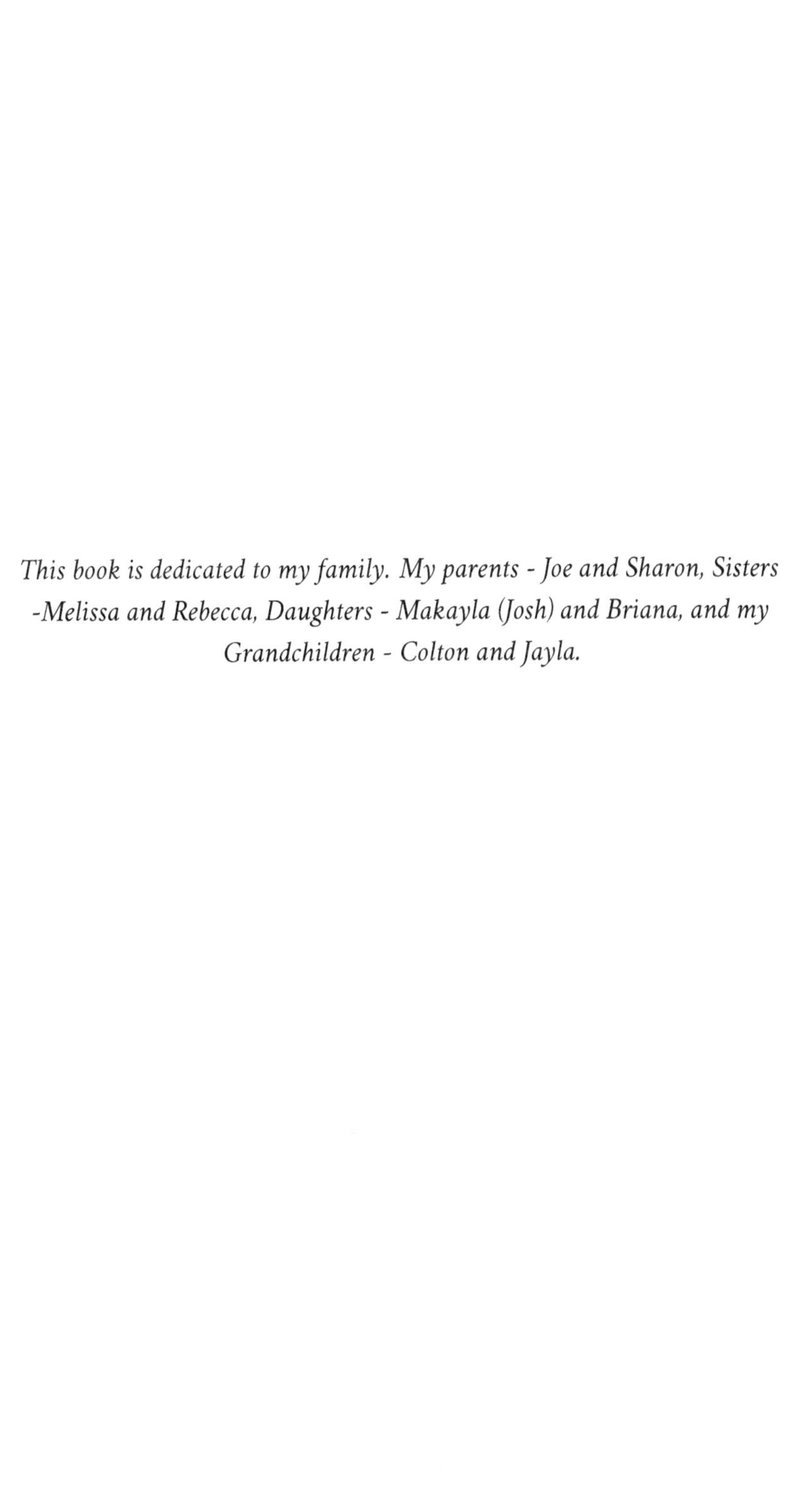

This book is dedicated to my family. My parents - Joe and Sharon, Sisters -Melissa and Rebecca, Daughters - Makayla (Josh) and Briana, and my Grandchildren - Colton and Jayla.

Contents

Introduction

I'm so excited you chose to explore "Live The Carnivore Diet Life". It's fun to share my Carnivore Journey and I hope you're able to find some incredible benefits as you begin yours. This book won't get into the science of why meat is amazing for your body, because there are people much more informed on that than I am.

I've learned so much from the likes of Scott Mys, Bella the Steak and Butter Girl, her coaches Emily and Raymond and Kelly Hogan to name a few. I will be eternally grateful for those who have gone against the powers-that-be to give us the knowledge about food that we deserve. I want to thank Dr. Ken Berry, Dr. Sean Baker, and Dr Elizabeth Bright for sharing their endless wisdom and knowledge on the carnivore lifestyle.

This book will get you started and give you the insight and information to confidently move forward in your own carnivore journey. Have fun with it and don't get too carried away with the "rules". There are so many variations and opinions out there so find a community where you are comfortable, eat your meat and start enjoying the many benefits!

1

How It All Started For Me

Before we dig into the meat and (not potatoes) of this book, I want to share a bit about my journey with the carnivore way of eating. We've had an on again-off again relationship. When I've been away from Carnivore my body is angry! That's why I know the carnivore diet will always be a part of my lifestyle.

Let's go back several years to my 40th year. I was walking and running several days a week, as a means to keep off the extra pounds. I began having intermittent hip pain and I convinced my chiropractor to take x-rays. She discovered some abnormalities in my hips. The ball joint on my right leg was twice the size as normal and was rotated at a 90 degree angle. Dr. Heidi referred me to a specialist in a nearby town to see what their recommendations would be.

When I presented my x-ray to the surgeon he immediately said, "I'll be replacing your hips before you turn 50". Now, if you know anything about me, you know that the statement he made kinda pissed me off! I tend to have a rebellious streak and don't like to be told I can't do something or that something is inevitable. Dr. Arrogant surgeon also told me that I have very shallow hip sockets which added to my problem. Without asking me a single question about my diet or lifestyle, he offered me a cortisone shot, which I declined, and he said I could follow-up when the pain got worse. Yep, that's it.

I decided to take matters into my own hands and prove him wrong. I knew a bit about inflammation and I began searching for ways to help combat it. Within a few weeks I had found the Ketogenic diet which I immediately adopted and was relieved from the discomfort in my hip in a matter of days. I stuck with the keto way of eating and was walking up to 20 miles a week without recurrent pain.

As the fall of 2019 approached, my oldest daughter was getting married and I wanted to drop some extra weight. I'd been listening to a podcast called, "Carnivore Cast" (now, called The Scott Mys Show). I decided I really wanted to give up the keto treats that I was addicted to and see if Carnivore would help release the extra weight. It did. I dropped about 30#s and felt great for the wedding. Because I didn't set a goal beyond the wedding, carbohydrate-laden foods started creeping back into my diet and I slowly faded from eating carnivore for a while.

Enter the fall of 2020. Life was CRAZY. Not just for the obvious world issues that were occurring, but also due to many other life events. My pregnant daughter, son-in-law, and grandson were all living in the basement while their house was built. In addition I was working from home and homeschooling my grandson. Stress levels were a tad high and my body freaked out. I developed a rash on my neck from right under my chin down to my upper chest. It was red, ugly and man, did it ever itch! And the former hip pain started popping back into my life. Oh goody.

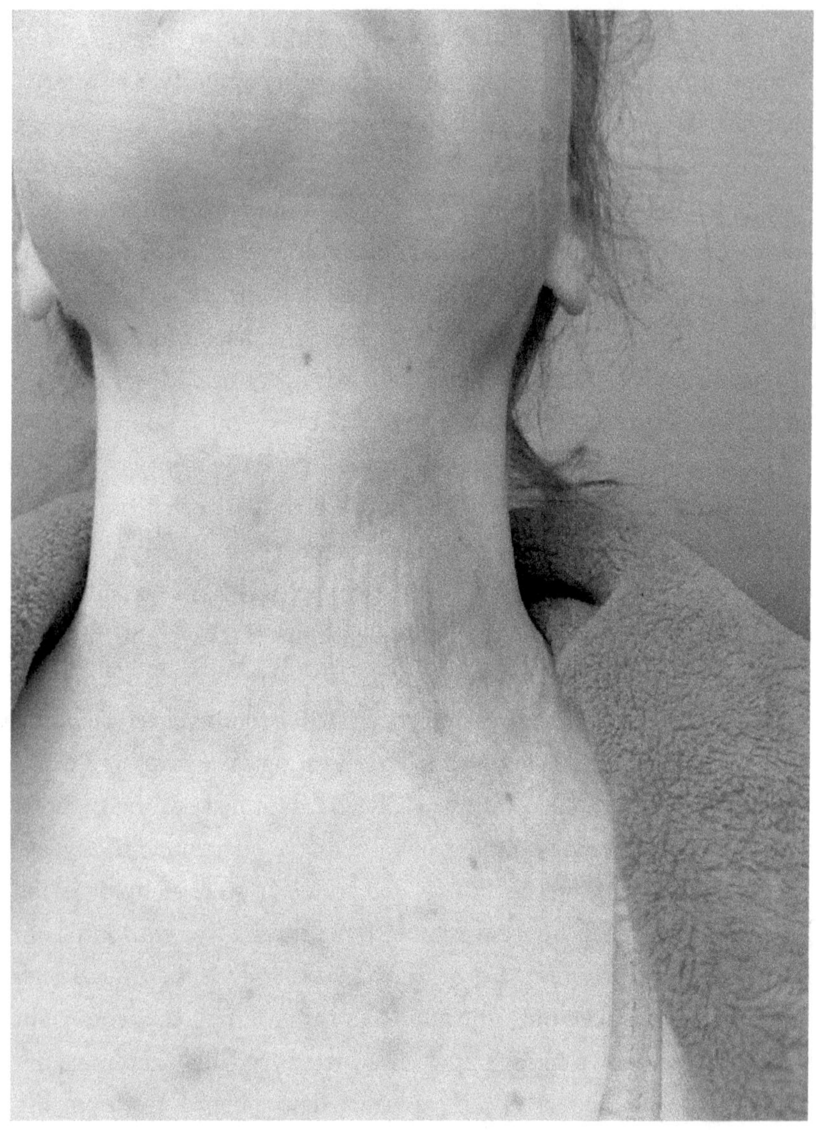

My neck fall of 2020

I'm a believer in natural health, so I tried all the supplements and essential oils I could think of with little success. I was several months into the rash and discomfort before my brain clicked and I remembered that there might be some benefit from returning to Carnivore. Again, there was. Within days the hip stopped aching, my neck stopped itching and the redness faded away.

As the years ticked away I dug deeper into carnivore diet podcasts and videos. I ate it up. I began to realize we have been duped into thinking that meat and butter are evil and that fruit and veggies are the perfect food for the body. I joined the Steak and Butter Gang and learned so much from the coaches and other members. Support is key when you start your journey. Especially if people in your life think you've lost your mind for eating only meat.

The final "stick it to the Dr." came in 2023 when I successfully thru-hiked the Appalachian trail in 6-months. That's walking 2,293.4 miles on my own feet and hips! I've learned how to eat to keep inflammation at bay. Thus, hip pain is absent when I live like a carnivore. I'm convinced that if I continue to eat mostly Carnivore, I will die without ever having to go through joint replacement surgery. I hope that you find a similar story for your life.

I don't want to bore you with a lot of ancient history on the topic, however, it is important to know that our ancestors ate meat. Think back to ancient times when people depended on livestock for survival. Cattle, sheep, and goats were treasured not only for their meat but also for milk, hides, and even helping with work.

Fast forward to medieval Europe, where the wealthy indulged in grand feasts filled with roasted meats, while common folk relied on preserved cuts or whatever they could hunt. Meat was seen as an essential part of a healthy diet, and when it was scarce, people often noticed their health declined. Similar stories about the importance of meat can be found worldwide: Indigenous peoples in the Americas used every part of the buffalo, and Asian cultures developed methods like curing and fermenting to make their meat last longer and go further.

As trade routes expanded and preservation methods improved, meat became more accessible to people of all classes. By the 19th and 20th centuries, inventions like refrigeration made it easier than ever to enjoy fresh meat regularly. Even with current debates about diet, meat has stood the test of time.

Why does the carnivore diet work: It's simple—our bodies thrive on whole, nutrient-dense foods, and nothing fits that description better than meat. By cutting out processed foods, sugars, and unnecessary carbs, you're giving your body a chance to reset and function the way it was designed to. With fewer of those inflammatory foods in your diet, you'll naturally shed weight, feel less bloated, and have more energy to do the things you love.

I've done all the diets, starting in about 7th grade with the Rice Diet. I didn't even need to be dieting because I wasn't overweight at that time. It consisted of no fat, lots of veggies and some rice. I was always hungry and my body was freezing cold. Now I understand why.

One of the biggest "Aha" moments that brought me to the carnivore diet came when I heard someone say that nurses often report that when changing colostomy bags on patients, undigested food was frequently found within the bags. Of course most people would assume that food was meat, because we've been told that meat will rot in your gut. Right? Wrong!

Nurses and individuals with colostomies often observe undigested food particles in their ostomy pouches, particularly from high-fiber foods like vegetables. This is because certain fibrous components of vegetables are resistant to complete digestion, leading to their presence in the output. In contrast, meat is generally well-digested, resulting in fewer visible remnants in colostomy output.

To me it just makes sense to eat the meat. Otherwise, I'm wasting my time and money eating vegetables if they're just going to come out the other end undigested and unused by my body. In addition I don't have to throw the veggies out because they are molding in the fridge, uneaten. Meat, on the other hand, *is* well digested, nutrient-dense, and can be used to support all parts of my body. It's loaded with the fat, protein and vitamins that leave me feeling amazing.

Who's this book for? This book is for **you** if you're overweight, tired of dieting, are always feeling hungry, are addicted to sugar and starchy foods, want to support your hormonal system or if you just want to take control of your own health and wellness. I've learned to take responsibility for my own body and what goes into it. If I'm the weirdo in the room who only eats meat, I'm ok with that.

2

The Problem With Modern Diets

L et's face it: modern diets are a mess. Everywhere you turn, there's a new fad promising to be the answer to all your problems. Yet somehow, we're more bloated, tired, and unhealthy than ever before. What gives? The answer lies in the way our food system has evolved—and not for the better.

How Processed Foods and Carbs Wreak Havoc on Your Body

It's a good policy to question what you've been told about what you should eat. The food pyramid,for example, has changed several times since I was a kid and yet we become fatter and fatter. Supposedly if we stick to what it shows we should eat, we'll all be healthy and fit. Is it really wise to stuff ourselves with the quantity of grains we're told to consume? Products including cereal, bread, chips, crackers and virtually all packaged foods are now designed to cause addiction. On top of that, our grains are sprayed with chemicals that have been proven to be harmful not only to the human body, but also to the environment.

Chemicals that are frequently sprayed onto fields include **Malathion**, **Aluminum Phosphide**, **Diazinon** and **Glyphosate**. Malathion is commonly used to kill fleas on our pets, treat head-lice infestations and to control garden insects. Aluminum Phosphide is commonly used on crop fields because it's an inexpensive way to control pests. It's been shown to affect tissues of the cardiac and vascular systems which can result in heart issues including cardiac failure. Diazinon is another common herbicide used in agriculture. Exposure to it has caused symptoms from headache and dizziness to anxiety, vision issues, respiratory difficulty and even coma. Glyphosate is commonly used on fields of corn, soy and wheat to kill unwanted weeds. Not only have these crops been genetically modified to be resistant to the glyphosate, but they are doused in a chemical that has been linked to up to a 41% increase in Non-Hodgkin Lymphoma.

We feed cereal, crackers and bread to our families and load them up with strawberries, carrots and spinach because it's "healthy." Consider how the foods were grown. The truth is we are trying to nourish our babies, kids and spouses and we are slowly poisoning them. That should disturb you and make you incredibly angry. If you want to be more informed about what you put in and on your body, start reading ingredient labels. I'm not talking about just food either. Pick an ingredient from the list on the back of the product and type "dangers of (ingredient)" into an on-line search engine. The results are quite eye-opening and often alarming. This problem is much deeper than one would think, and that might require another book.

The food industry employs various strategies to make their products more appealing and to encourage increased consumption. One method they employ is the use of the "bliss point," a term coined by market researcher Howard Moskowitz. This concept refers to the precise combination of sugar, salt, and fat that maximizes a food's palatability, making it more enjoyable and potentially leading to over consumption. That's what the food industry wants because if we eat more, their pockets grow thicker. And we get fatter and sicker.

Additionally, companies invest in exploring *sensory experiences* associated with their products. Techniques such as sonic branding—designing specific sounds like the crunch of a chip or the fizz of a soda can—are crafted to trigger cravings and reinforce brand recognition. By manipulating aromas, companies can attract consumers and encourage repeat purchases. These aromas or chemicals are additionally contributing to the decline of health and the increase of disease.

Have you ever noticed how hard it is to stop at just one chip or a single cookie? That's no accident. As I mentioned previously, processed foods are carefully designed to keep you coming back for more. They're loaded with sugar, refined carbs, and artificial ingredients that mess with your body's natural signals. Instead of feeling full and satisfied, you end up craving even more junk.

What's worse, these foods wreak havoc on your blood sugar levels. A bowl of oatmeal, cereal or a sugary granola bar might give you a quick burst of energy, but it's always followed by a crash. And that crash leaves you reaching for another snack, or more coffee to get through the day. It's a vicious cycle that leads to weight gain, inflammation, and a bunch of other health problems like obesity, diabetes, and cardiovascular diseases. .

That's why I am so excited about the next four years and the future of the food industry. I hold great hope that good things are coming to our tables and thus to the lives of my family and my fellow Americans.

Common Health Issues: Belly Fat, Bloating, Aches, and Fatigue

If you're like most people, you've probably dealt with at least one of these issues. Maybe it's that stubborn belly fat that won't budge, no matter how many crunches you do. Or maybe you've had those afternoons where you're so bloated you can barely button your pants. It's not just uncomfortable—it's your body's way of telling you something is wrong. Perhaps you're even dealing with skin issues or something more significant like disease.

Processed foods and carb-heavy diets are a big part of the problem. They cause inflammation in your gut, which can lead to bloating and digestive discomfort. And that inflammation doesn't just stop at your stomach. It can contribute to aches, pains (my hip pain), and even chronic fatigue. Your body is literally crying out for help. You tell your doctor and out comes the prescription pad. But that's a whole other topic that I might get into some other time!

Why Other Diets Often Fail

Here's the truth: most diets are too complicated. They're full of rules, restrictions, and tiny portions that leave you hungry and frustrated. Counting calories, tracking macros, and meal prepping every day might work for some people, but for most of us? It's not sustainable.

The other issue is that many diets don't address the root cause of the problem. They focus on cutting calories or avoiding fat without considering the quality of the food you're eating. You can't outsmart your body with low-fat cookies or diet soda. Those foods might save you a few calories in the short term, but they're still loaded with the same addictive, inflammatory ingredients that got you into trouble in the first place.

That's where the carnivore diet comes in. It's simple, satisfying, and effective because it eliminates the junk and focuses on real, nourishing food. No calorie counting. No complicated meal plans. Just eating the way your body was designed to thrive.

3

What is the Carnivore Diet?

I f you've ever wished for a diet that doesn't come with a mile-long list of rules, the carnivore diet might be your dream come true. It's as straightforward as it gets: eat meat. That's it. No need for calorie counting, macro tracking, or stressing about whether a handful of almonds will ruin your progress. I simply love how easy this way of life is and I have certainly tailored it to my needs and way of life. You will learn to do the same thing.

The Simplicity of Eating Only Animal-Based Foods

At its core, the carnivore diet is all about keeping things simple. You're cutting out all the extras—the grains, the veggies, the sugars, the processed junk—and sticking to nutrient-dense, animal-based foods. This includes beef, chicken, pork, fish, eggs, and even butter and cheese (if your body handles dairy well). I'll provide a comprehensive list of things I eat. Many carnivores also like to include raw dairy if it's available. You may have to get on-line and look for local herd-shares to

12

have access to it, as it's heavily regulated at this time.

Think about it: our ancestors didn't have snack bars, cereal, or frozen pizzas at their fingertips. They thrived on what they could hunt or gather, and meat was often the centerpiece of their diet. The carnivore diet takes this idea and makes it accessible for everyone.

Why Less is More When it Comes to Your Food Choices

One of the best parts of the carnivore diet is how freeing it feels. Instead of standing in the grocery store aisle, overwhelmed by a hundred different options, you can skip the noise and head straight to the meat section. Your meals don't need to be fancy or complicated to be satisfying.

And here's the thing: by cutting out all the extras, you're giving your body a break. No more buying a laundry list of ingredients or wondering why that "healthy" granola bar left you bloated. You're focusing on foods that your body knows how to process and use efficiently. My meals are quite often one single item which doesn't require a pile of pots, pans and a bunch of clean-up. I love that!

A Diet That Works With Your Body, Not Against It

Here's a little secret: when you eat the right foods, your body takes care of the rest. The carnivore diet works because it gives your body exactly what it needs: high-quality protein and fat. These are the building blocks for energy, muscle repair, and all the other amazing things your body does every day.

When you're eating meat, you're naturally fueling your body in a way that feels satisfying. There's no blood sugar crash a couple of hours later, no gnawing hunger that makes you raid the pantry at midnight. Just steady, reliable energy and a feeling of fullness that lasts. When you're hungry, just eat. By eating meat and animal products the cravings for sugar quickly fade and cravings for more meat increase.

The carnivore diet is about getting back to basics and letting your body do what it was designed to do: ***thrive***.

The Lion Diet: An Even Simpler Approach

If you're ready to take simplicity to the next level, there's the Lion Diet. It's a highly restrictive version of the carnivore diet that focuses solely on ruminant animals (like beef, lamb, and goat), salt, and water. That's it. The Lion Diet is often used as an elimination diet to identify food sensitivities or to help with severe autoimmune issues. By stripping down your food choices even further, you give your body a chance to heal and reset. The amazing thing about the human body is the God-given ability to heal. When we remove all foods that are making it sick, the body can function as it was designed to. It's not for everyone, but for those who need a complete dietary reset, the Lion Diet can be a game-changer. Mikhaila Peterson is the gal to follow with super knowledge in this way of eating. She even has a Ted Talk that I highly recommend.

4

Benefits of the Carnivore Diet

The carnivore diet offers more than just a new way of eating—it can transform your health and quality of life. Let's dive into the many benefits this meat-focused lifestyle can bring.

1. Weight Loss Without Counting Calories

One of the biggest perks of the carnivore diet is effortless weight loss for many people. By eliminating carbs and focusing on protein and fat, your body naturally shifts into fat-burning mode called ketosis. Studies have shown that high-protein diets help regulate hunger hormones, meaning you'll feel full longer and eat less without even trying.

2. Reduced Inflammation

Chronic inflammation is at the root of many health issues, including joint pain, autoimmune diseases, and heart problems. The carnivore diet cuts out inflammatory foods like sugar, seed oils, and grains. Instead, it provides anti-inflammatory nutrients like omega-3s and conjugated linoleic acid (CLA) found in fatty meats. The speed at which I experienced joint pain relief still blows my mind.

3. Improved Digestion

If you've struggled with bloating, IBS, or food intolerances, the carnivore diet can be a game-changer. Meat is highly bioavailable, meaning your body digests it easily and absorbs its nutrients efficiently. Many people report relief from stomach issues within days of switching to carnivore. Over time you may find that gas is eliminated and bowel movements become less "fragrant". I struggled with constipation my entire childhood and well into my 30s, however, that is no longer an issue with the carnivore life.

4. Steady Energy Levels

Say goodbye to energy crashes and constant snacking. On the carnivore diet, your body uses fat as its primary fuel source, which provides a steady stream of energy throughout the day. Without blood sugar spikes and dips, you'll feel more alert and focused. Many carnivores show increased energy levels within days of starting the carnivore diet.

5. Enhanced Mental Clarity

A diet rich in animal-based nutrients can do wonders for your brain. Omega-3 fatty acids, vitamin B12, and zinc—all abundant in meat—support cognitive function and mental clarity. Frequently people on the carnivore diet report feeling sharper and more focused.

6. Relief from Autoimmune Symptoms

For those with autoimmune conditions, the carnivore diet can offer significant relief. By eliminating plant-based triggers like lectins, oxalates, and gluten, many people see reductions in symptoms like joint pain, skin issues, and fatigue. This elimination approach allows your body to heal and reset.

7. Easier Meal Planning

Let's face it: life is busy, and complicated meal prep can be a hassle. The carnivore diet is as simple as it gets. With just a few ingredients—meat, salt, and fat—you can whip up satisfying meals in no time. It's perfect for those who want a no-fuss approach to eating.

8. A Happier Relationship with Food

On the carnivore diet, you'll ditch the diet culture mindset of counting calories, obsessing over macros and measuring or weighing your food. Instead, you'll learn to listen to your body's hunger and satiety signals. Eating becomes a joyful and intuitive experience, free from guilt or restriction.

9. Clearer Skin

Skin conditions like acne, eczema, and rosacea often improve on the carnivore diet. Removing processed foods and potential allergens gives your body the chance to heal from the inside out. Many people notice a natural glow and fewer breakouts within weeks.

10. Improved Sleep

Eating nutrient-dense foods like meat and avoiding sugar can have a profound impact on your sleep quality. High-protein diets are linked to deeper, more restorative sleep—so you'll wake up feeling refreshed and ready to tackle the day.

11. Sexual Health

The carnivore diet may enhance sexual health by improving hormone balance, boosting energy, and promoting overall vitality. Here's how it works:

The Carnivore Diet Supports Hormone Regulation
1. **Increased Testosterone**: Cholesterol and saturated fat in meat are essential for producing sex hormones, including testosterone. Higher testosterone levels can improve libido, mood, and sexual performance in both men and women.
2. **Balanced Hormones for Women** -The Carnivore Diet may:

- ***Regulate insulin and estrogen,*** due to the elimination of processed foods and sugars, which helps reduce hormonal imbalances that might interfere with sexual health.
- ***Improve Circulation*** - Healthy blood flow is crucial for sexual function. Nutrient-dense foods like red meat and fatty fish provide omega-3 fatty acids and nitric oxide precursors, which support vascular health and improve circulation.
- ***Reduce Inflammation*** - Chronic inflammation is linked to conditions like erectile dysfunction (ED) and low libido. By removing inflammatory foods such as grains, seed oils, and sugar, the carnivore diet helps reduce inflammation and supports better sexual function.
- ***Enhance Energy and Stamina*** - Stable energy levels on the carnivore diet lead to improved physical stamina. Without sugar crashes or carb-induced fatigue, people often find they have more endurance and vitality.
- ***Boost Mental Clarity and Mood*** - Sexual health isn't just physical; it's mental too. Nutrients like zinc, vitamin B12, and iron, which are abundant in meat, support brain health and can reduce anxiety or stress that may impact libido.
- ***Improve Overall Confidence*** - Weight loss, better body composition, and increased energy on the carnivore diet can boost self-esteem,

which plays a significant role in a healthy sex life. By focusing on nutrient-dense, whole foods and eliminating inflammatory triggers, the carnivore diet creates a foundation for better sexual health and overall well-being.

$$5$$

Getting Started with the Carnivore Diet

You likely picked up this book because you heard about the benefits of a carnivore lifestyle that connected with you. With a little preparation and the right mindset, you'll be on your way to reaping the benefits in no time. Here's how to set yourself up for success.

Preparing Your Kitchen and Mindset

First things first: let's get your kitchen ready. Say goodbye to the carbs and processed snacks that tempt you. Clear out the pantry and fridge of anything that doesn't align with your new way of eating. Really commit to this. If you leave snacks and food for others, you're setting yourself up for temptation, only making things harder for yourself. Maybe this is a bit harder if you have a spouse who refuses to eat only meat, but I would try to come up with a compromise. Perhaps gather all the foods that they want to keep eating and put them in a single cupboard that you just don't open. When you have cleared out the garbage-foods, you have your clean slate.

But it's not just about your kitchen—you need the right mindset, too. Understand that the first few weeks might come with some challenges as your body adjusts. Stay committed and remind yourself why you're doing this. The long-term benefits are worth it. This is the time to reach out to others who have adopted the same lifestyle. On social media, join an existing group like Steak and Butter Gang or follow any other carnivore influencer that you connect with. This community is amazing and you'll find the right fit for you. Clear out the negative thoughts and replace them with positive affirmations like, "I'm so proud of the changes I'm making for my health", or "I'm focusing on one good choice at a time". Kick the lies of the enemy to the curb and focus on where you are heading.

What to Eat: Meat and Animal-Based Products

The carnivore diet is straightforward. Your main focus is meat, and lots of it. Think steaks, burgers, chicken thighs, pork chops, and fish. You can also enjoy eggs, butter, and even some dairy, like cheese or cream if your body can handle it. Simplicity is the name of the game, so don't stress about variety. When first starting, give yourself grace with the meats you choose. I choose to include sausages, bacon, brats, nitrate-free lunch meats and a few other slightly processed meats. The key is to make it easy to reach for something carnivore-friendly when hunger strikes. Become a consumer of ingredient lists and choose no-sugar items. Even small amounts of sugar and sweeteners can prevent you from removing the sugar/carb cravings.

Here's a pro tip: choose fatty cuts of meat whenever possible and eat that first. Fat is your friend on this diet, providing energy and helping you stay full longer. Ribeyes, ground beef with higher fat content, and pork belly are all great options. I usually cook my meat in an air fryer to develop a beautiful crust on the outside and the perfect "doneness" on the inside. The one I use is the Tastee brand air fryer because it's PFOA/PFOS-free and the temperature setting goes higher than (450 degrees) most other air-fryers.

Other methods I use when preparing meals include grilling, baking, crockpot cooking, and stove top methods. Use any form of cooking that you prefer to keep yourself well fed and happy.

Here's a list of foods I consume on the carnivore diet.

Beef (consider purchasing a ¼, ½, or whole beef for better pricing. Also, get to know local farmers and you'll have a better idea of how the animal was raised)

1. Steaks
2. Roast
3. Burger - patties, browned, meatballs
4. Ribs
5. Stew Meat
6. Fat/tallow
7. Organs if desired (I don't)

Pork

- Sausage
- Pork Belly
- Pork Booty
- Ribs
- Chops
- Ham (watch for sugar)
- Bacon (watch for sugar)

- Pork Rinds

Chicken

- Thighs
- Wings
- Breast (limited due to no fat)
- Canned chicken (for Meatzza)

Other Meats

- Venison - I often pressure-can mine. It makes a quick, take-along meal in a jar.
- Lamb
- Goat
- Rabbit
- Bison
- Salami
- Pepperoni
- Brats
- Hot Dogs
- Fish

Dairy & Eggs

- Cheese
- Cream Cheese
- Cottage Cheese
- Parmesan
- Butter
- Ghee

- Plain Greek Yogurt (full fat)
- Heavy Cream
- Sour Cream
- Eggs - scrambled, fried, poached or boiled

Realize that this is **not** an all-inclusive list. It's what I choose to eat. You may find that you like organ meats, so by all means, include those. I also drink tea, carbonated water and coffee. I like to include sugar-free seasonings and spices in some meals as well. Do what works for you within the simple guidelines and you will be just fine. You will likely adjust your eating style as you progress in this way of life. This is simply a starting point to aim you in the direction of better health.

What to Avoid: Hidden Carbs and Processed Foods

This part is crucial: avoid any foods that sneak in hidden carbs or processed ingredients. That means sauces, marinades, or seasonings that include sugar or starch should not be used. When in doubt, keep it plain and simple. Salt is your best friend, and it's all you really need to bring out the flavor of your meals. If you really need something on top, I'll give you an option in the 7-day meal plan in the next chapter.

Processed foods, even ones labeled as "keto" or "paleo," are often loaded with ingredients that don't align with the carnivore diet. Stick to whole, unprocessed animal-based foods, and you'll be good.

6

Meal Plans and Tips

Sample 7-Day Meal Plan

Getting started can feel daunting, so here's a simple 7-day meal plan to guide you. Each day includes three meals, but feel free to adjust based on your hunger levels. And if you're really hungry, have a carnivore snack like jerky, cottage cheese or beef sticks.

Day 1:

- Breakfast: 3-4 scrambled eggs cooked in butter, 3-4 slices of bacon.
- Lunch: Grilled ribeye steak with a pat of butter.
- Dinner: Pan-seared salmon with crispy chicken skin on the side.

Day 2:

- Breakfast: Omelet with 4 eggs and diced ham, cooked in tallow.
- Lunch: Ground beef patties topped with melted cheddar cheese.
- Dinner: Pork belly strips with a side of bone broth.

Day 3:

- Breakfast: 2-4 sunny-side-up eggs and a sausage link or two.
- Lunch: Rotisserie chicken (dark meat preferred) with crispy skin.
- Dinner: Lamb chops cooked in ghee with salt to taste.

Day 4:

- Breakfast: Steak and eggs Choose your own size and quantity.
- Lunch: Grilled shrimp with melted butter for dipping.
- Dinner: Roast beef with a side of bone broth.

Day 5:

- Breakfast: 4 hard-boiled eggs and a slice or two of cheddar cheese.
- Lunch: Pan-fried chicken thighs seasoned with salt.
- Dinner: Taco bowl (seasoned beef, shredded cheese, sour cream)

Day 6:

- Breakfast: 3-4 poached eggs with a drizzle of melted butter.
- Lunch: Grilled pork ribs with salt, pepper and Bacon Mayo (below).
- Dinner: Baked salmon topped with garlic butter.

Day 7:

- Breakfast: Bacon-wrapped sausage links with a side of scrambled eggs.
- Lunch: Turkey drumstick cooked in its own juices.
- Dinner: Slow-cooked beef short ribs, fall-off-the-bone tender.

Bonus Recipe: I love pizza and this is my fallback when I get the craving.

Meatzza

Crust:

1 - 12.5oz can chicken

½ c. canned parmesan cheese

1 egg

Toppings:

Mozzarella cheese plus your choice of meat toppings such as pepperoni, ham salami, shredded chicken, sausage or any leftover meats on hand.

Combine chicken, parmesan and egg. Mix with a fork.

Place a piece of parchment paper on a baking pan or stoneware pizza dish.

Spread chicken mixture on pan and spread into desired shape.

Bake @ 375 degrees fahrenheit for 25-30 min.

Sprinkle with Mozzarella and add meat toppings.

Sprinkle a bit more Mozzarella and some Parmesan if desired.

Bake for an additional 15-20 minutes.

Remove from the oven and enjoy!

Bacon Mayo

2 egg yolks (you can add the whites to scrambled eggs or to bread chicken with

crushed pork rinds for another meal)

2 tsp water

1 cup bacon grease or reserved meat drippings

½ tsp salt

⅛ tsp garlic powder (optional)

Add all ingredients to a tall glass or jar. Using an immersion blender, slowly raise and lower the blender until the mixture emulsifies. It will be a similar texture to what you used to buy in the store. Use immediately or store in the refrigerator for up to a week.

If you don't have an immersion blender you can also use a mini blender to get the same result.

Creative Ideas for Eating on the Go

Here are a few tips to keep your meals carnivore-friendly while out and about:

1. Portable Protein: Pack hard-boiled eggs, jerky (without sugar or additives), or pork rinds for easy snacking.
2. Fast Food Hacks: Order burger patties without the bun or sauces and add extra cheese or bacon.
3. Canned Options: Stock up on canned sardines, tuna, or salmon for a quick and easy meal. Also, consider pressure canning meat for an amazing convenient meal.
4. Deli Counter Finds: Grab sliced roast beef, turkey, or other meats (just check for added sugars).
5. Travel-Friendly Fat: Bring small containers of butter, ghee, or tallow to add to meals for extra flavor and satiety.

I learned how to make pemmican with different meats and tallow I rendered from the beef I purchased. It takes a bit of effort to get to the end result, but the effort is definitely over-shadowed by the reward. It is a high fat fuel to keep you satisfied and full of energy. It's one of my favorite foods to pack for hiking.

Managing Social Situations

Eating like a carnivore doesn't mean you have to become a hermit. Continue to live your life with a few simple changes. Here are some ideas to navigate social settings:

1. Host a Meat Feast: If you're in charge, grill up steaks, burgers, or ribs for everyone to enjoy. You can have cheese and sausage trays as well.

2. Eat Ahead: Have a filling meal before heading out to a restaurant to avoid temptation. Restaurant meals are often not as filling without breaking the bank, so by eating a small meal at home first, you won't get left feeling unsatisfied and then be tempted to eat something you regret later.

3. Simplify Your Order: At restaurants, stick to steak, burgers, or grilled chicken, and ask for no sauces or sides. My standard is a burger patty or two topped with bacon, cheese and mustard.

4. Explain if Needed: If someone asks about why you're eating this way, keep it simple: "I feel best when I stick to meat-based meals" or "I eat low-carb to help reduce inflammation in my hip." It's becoming more common and less strange for people to hear about these choices.

5. Bring Your Own: For potlucks or gatherings, bring a carnivore-friendly dish or two, like meatballs or a roast. Meat trays filled with deli meats and cheeses are always a good bet too and are often the first thing people go for.

7

Overcoming Challenges

E mbarking on the carnivore diet can be rewarding, but it's not without its bumps along the way. Here's how to tackle some common challenges you may find early on in your journey.

Adapting to the Diet

Let's talk about the transition phase. For most people, the first week or two can be a bit rocky. You might experience what's known as the "keto flu" with symptoms like fatigue, headaches, or cravings as your body adapts to burning fat for fuel instead of carbs. This is completely normal and temporary. Hopefully this phase is not part of your journey and you can simply move along.

To ease the transition, make sure you're drinking plenty of water and adding salt to your meals. Electrolytes (salts) are your secret weapon during this phase. We've been told for years that salt is bad for you, but it's another thing I learned to question the narrative on. I've done my research and now liberally add salt to my foods, often before and after cooking. My favorite salts are Redmond Real Salt, Baja Gold Mineral Sea Salt and Selina Naturally Celtic Sea Salt.

Don't forget to eat enough! One of the biggest mistakes new carnivores make is not eating enough food. Give yourself permission to dig into that extra steak or add a couple more eggs to your breakfast. Your body has actually been starved of nutrition for a long time and now you're going to have to make up for that. Eating more meat will help your body repair and keep you feeling full longer. If you're hungry, eat meat. If you're craving sweets, eat meat. It really truly is that easy. As you begin this journey you may want to eat 3 meals a day. Perhaps a snack or two as well. It's ok. Do it. The way you live like a carnivore will change and progress over time and that's the beauty of it. One day you might look at the clock and realize it's 5pm and you haven't eaten yet, and you're not even that hungry. It still blows my mind when this happens.

The transition phase is just a small hurdle on your journey. Stick with it, and soon you'll start to feel incredible benefits—more energy, better digestion, and a sense of freedom from constant hunger and cravings. It took years to get where you currently are, so be patient with yourself. You've got this!

Dealing with Social Pressure

Explaining your diet to friends and family can be tough. Keep it simple: "This is what works best for my health." You don't owe anyone a detailed explanation, but if they're curious, share your experiences with enthusiasm and positivity. If they try to shame you or say they fear for your health you can share information with them in order to educate, or simply thank them for their concern and move on. Point them in the direction of Dr. Paul Salidino, Dr. Sean Baker, or Dr. Elizabeth Bright or one of the many other professionals involved with the carnivore community. And, you can always loan them this book when they see the light.

Staying Motivated

We are definitely a culture of people who want instant gratification, however, results might not come overnight. Track your progress with photos, measurements, or a journal to remind yourself of the improvements you're making. Celebrate small wins, like clearer skin, better sleep, or improved energy. Try to put the scale away and notice how you feel after a few days, a week, a month and so on. The scale is not your friend. Especially on a carnivore journey. You will notice smaller clothing sizes much sooner than you will see a change in the scale. Your body will be recompositioning and changing. Trust the process and you will love the result. I encourage keeping a journal in your first few months. Write down minor changes you're noticing and you'll be amazed down the road at just how far you have come.

8

Carnivore Diet and Exercise

Fueling your body with meat and an active lifestyle can go hand in hand. I hiked many miles along Michigan's North Country Scenic Trail on a meat heavy diet and felt amazing. Here's how the carnivore diet can fit into your fitness routine:

Energy and Performance

Once your body adapts to using fat for fuel, you may find you have more stable energy throughout the day, making workouts feel more sustainable and less taxing. You'll likely notice improved recovery times as well. During your first month or two however, try to avoid new fitness routines and hard workouts. Your body will be adjusting and by giving it a loving rest you will likely start feeling the desire to get up and move.

Walking is a fantastic form of movement that you can take on from day one and I highly encourage it. After you eat a meal, it's a great idea to go for a little walk. Especially if you think you might want to eat more after your meal. The walk will give your body time to "think" about what you consumed. Afterward, if you're still hungry, then by all means, have another burger.

Types of Exercise

The carnivore diet supports a variety of activities, from strength training to cardio. Whether you're hitting the weights, going for a jog, or hiking local trails, animal-based foods provide the nutrients your muscles need to perform and recover. Whatever physical activity makes you happy, then that's what you should do.

Staying Fueled

You may need to do a little experimenting when it comes to working out. Some people find they perform much better if they wait to eat until after they exercise. However, if you are dragging and just don't have the energy, then try a small meal before the workout. Stick to a simple meal like a steak or some ground beef. Post-workout, replenish with fatty cuts of meat or a few eggs to help your muscles repair and grow.

9

Traveling on Carnivore

Staying carnivore while traveling for work or vacations might seem challenging, but it's completely doable with a bit of planning. And that planning will be key to your success.

Packing Essentials

Bring portable snacks like beef jerky (unsweetened), pork rinds, or canned sardines. Hard-boiled eggs and small containers of butter or ghee can also come in handy. Cheese travels well and you can now find many individual size options in the store. Karen Miles, a carnivore peer, takes bacon in a baggie when she goes out and it's become known as "purse bacon". Who knew that was a thing?

Eating Out

Most restaurants have carnivore-friendly options. Order steaks, burgers (hold the bun), or grilled chicken. Skip sauces and sides, and ask for extra butter, sour cream or cheese if needed. You can call the

35

restaurant ahead of time and ask about what oils they use for cooking and if you are able to make special requests such as not cooking your meat in seed oils. Most restaurants are very familiar with food allergies and sensitivities and will accommodate your requests.

Hotel Stays

If your hotel has a mini-fridge, stock it with deli meats, smoked salmon, or pre-cooked bacon. A travel-sized electric grill or hot plate can make cooking simple meals in your room easy. One of my favorite ways to get extra fat while I'm traveling is to take my mini blender and pop a tablespoon or two of butter into my morning coffee. It turns into a delightful frothy drink that I adore. If you're not a coffee drinker, try this trick with beef or chicken broth. Use some caution with the liquid butter as some people experience stomach upset.

10

Monitoring Your Progress

Tracking your progress on the carnivore diet is key to staying motivated and making adjustments as needed. I'm not talking about tracking as in counting carbs or calories or measuring your food. I'm talking about tracking your body and how it changes, as well as your mental health and moods. It's really easy to forget how we've changed on the physical and mental side of things.

What to Track
- Physical Changes: Take photos and measure your waist, hips, and other key areas to monitor fat loss.
- Health Improvements: Note changes in digestion, energy levels, sleep quality, or chronic pain.
- Mental Clarity: Many people report improved focus and reduced brain fog.

Adjusting Your Approach

If you're not seeing the results you want, you can tweak your diet. Try incorporating more fatty cuts, reducing dairy, or experimenting with meal timing. Everyone's body is different, so it might take a little time to find your groove. If you really want to see what your body is sensitive to, it might be time to explore the Lion Diet that I mentioned earlier.

11

Long-Term Success

The carnivore diet isn't a short-term fix—it can be a sustainable way of life. You'll find people in the community that have been eating this way for 5, 10 and even 20+ years and are strong, healthy and feeling amazing. Here's how to make it work for the long haul:

Embracing Simplicity

Keep your meals simple and satisfying. Over time, you'll find that cravings for non-carnivore foods fade, and your body thrives on this way of eating. Keep meals simple and don't feel like you need to have a well rounded plate. One or two items on the plate are perfectly fine. If you get bored look for a new cookbook to get creative ideas from long-term carnivores.

Finding Your Routine

Stick to what works for you. Maybe that means meal prepping on

Sundays or rotating a few favorite meals to keep things easy. The key is consistency. This lifestyle is so simple it will blow your mind. All the years of counting calories, weighing your food and measuring out portions are a thing of the past. Find what works for you and you've got it made.

Staying Flexible

Life happens, and there may be times when you can't stick to the diet perfectly. That's okay. Focus on getting back on track with your <u>next</u> meal and remember how far you've come. Don't use a mistake as an excuse to gorge on every food known to man. Simply decide that the next meal will be a carnivore meal. You've got this. I'm so excited for you to experience all that Living Like A Carnivore will do for you!

12

Conclusion

Congratulations! By now, you've explored the ins and outs of the carnivore diet, from understanding its benefits and tackling common myths to practical tips for meals, social situations, and staying committed. The carnivore lifestyle isn't just about eating meat—it's about reclaiming your health, energy, and confidence in a way that feels natural and sustainable.

The journey to better health starts with small, intentional choices. Maybe you'll begin by swapping out carb-heavy meals for a satisfying steak, or perhaps you'll dive in headfirst and experience the full transformation. Either way, every step you take brings you closer to a life free of bloating, joint pain, and energy crashes—and filled with vitality, mental clarity, and a renewed sense of well-being.

Remember, this is *your* journey. The carnivore diet can be adapted to fit your needs, whether you're tackling health challenges, aiming to shed weight, or simply striving to feel your best. Be patient with yourself as you adjust to this new way of eating, and don't hesitate to experiment to find what works best for your body.

Most importantly, celebrate the wins. Notice the moments when your energy lasts all day, when your body feels stronger, or when you realize you've left behind food cravings that used to control you. Those moments are proof that you're making meaningful progress.

The carnivore diet may be unconventional, but it's rooted in a timeless truth: our bodies thrive when we fuel them with real, nutrient-dense food. By embracing this lifestyle, you're honoring your body and taking charge of your health in a powerful, transformative way.

Here's to living the carnivore life—and to a healthier, more energetic you!

If you've found any value from this book please give it a favorable review on Amazon right now so others can benefit too.

Follow my hiking adventures on YouTube @backpack and bible

13

Resources

iving with an Ostomy – Health Information Library | PeaceHealth. (n.d.). https://www.peacehealth.org/medical-topics/id/ug21 86?utm_source=chatgpt.com

Coloplast. (n.d.). *Coloplast.* https://www.coloplast.us/ostomy/peo ple-with-an-ostomy/living-with-a-stoma/food-and-beverage/?utm_ source=chatgpt.com

MOAP:: Nutritional Guidelines:: Colostomy. (n.d.). https://miami ostomyaftercare.org/Ostomy.php?op=NGO_Colostomy

Kumar, A. (2023, November 22). *Nutrition while living with an ostomy bag.* Uncancer LLC. https://www.uncancer.com/blogs/ news/nutrition-while-living-with-an-ostomy-bag

IARC Monograph on Glyphosate. (n.d.). https://www.iarc.who.int/feat ured-news/media-centre-iarc-news-glyphosate/

Malathion | ToxFAQsTM | ATSDR. (n.d.). https://wwwn.cdc.gov/TSP/ ToxFAQs/ToxFAQsDetails.aspx?faqid=521&toxid=92

Glyphosate herbicides and your health. (2024, June 24). WebMD. https://www.webmd.com/cancer/herbicide-glyphosate-cancer

Diazinon | Public Health Statement | ATSDR. (n.d.). https://wwwn.cdc.

gov/TSP/PHS/PHS.aspx?phsid=511&toxid=90

Gurjar, M., Baronia, A., Azim, A., & Sharma, K. (2011). Managing aluminum phosphide poisonings. *Journal of Emergencies Trauma and Shock, 4*(3), 378. https://doi.org/10.4103/0974-2700.83868

Schewitz, K. (2024, July 25). *A scientist who used to advise ultra-processed food companies shares 2 surprising ways they make food irresistible.* Business Insider. https://www.businessinsider.com/scientist-shares-how-companies-make-ultra-processed-foods-irresistible-2024-7?utm_source=chatgpt.com

Living with an Ostomy – Health Information Library | PeaceHealth. (n.d.-c). https://www.peacehealth.org/medical-topics/id/ug2186?utm_source=chatgpt.com

Wikipedia contributors. (2024, August 18). *Bliss point (food).* Wikipedia. https://en.wikipedia.org/wiki/Bliss_point_%28food%29?utm_source=chatgpt.com

Miller, K. (2024, December 19). Can You Actually Be Addicted to Ultra-Processed Snacks? Here's What the Science Says. *Health.* https://www.health.com/lawsuit-ultra-processed-foods-addictive-8762798?utm_source=chatgpt.com

General Resources Referenced:

Scientific Journals and Research

Studies on low-carbohydrate and ketogenic diets, their effects on inflammation, hormone regulation, and energy levels.

Research on high-protein diets and their impacts on satiety and weight loss.

Books and Authors on the Carnivore Diet

Shawn Baker's *The Carnivore Diet* for insights into practical application and benefits.

Paul Saladino's *The Carnivore Code* for information on nutrient density and inflammation reduction.

Diet and Nutrition Websites

Articles from PubMed, ScienceDirect, and similar platforms regarding the physiological impacts of a meat-based diet.

Blogs and forums like ZeroCarbZen, MeatRx (now Revero), and Carnivore Cast for anecdotal experiences and tips.

Personal Stories and Community Insights

Testimonials from individuals following carnivore or ketogenic diets, particularly related to energy, mental clarity, and sexual health.

Historical and Anthropological Contexts

Research on traditional meat-based diets in indigenous populations.

Food Industry and Addictive Foods

Investigative journalism pieces and books like Michael Moss's *Salt Sugar Fat: How the Food Giants Hooked Us.*

Research on food processing, artificial flavoring, and consumer behavior.

Nutritional Biochemistry

Information on the roles of micronutrients (e.g., zinc, B12, omega-3 fatty acids) in physical and mental health.

Data on bioavailability and digestion of animal-based versus plant-based nutrients.